# Tantric Sex

*The Ultimate Guide to Ignite Your Sex Life through Tantric Techniques*

# Table of Contents

# Introduction

Congratulations on purchasing your personal copy of *Tantric Sex*. Thank you for doing so.

The following chapters will discuss some of the many benefits and the history of tantra and tantric sex.

You will discover how important this practice can be to your well-being and your relationship with you partner.

The final chapter will explore how to practice tantric breathing to help prolong your sexual experience.

There are plenty of books on this subject on the market, thanks again for choosing this one! Every effort was made to ensure it is full of as much useful information as possible. Please enjoy!

Congratulations on purchasing your personal copy of *Tantric Sex*. Thank you for doing so.

# Tantric Sex

Tantric sex has been around for more than 5,000 years. It is an ancient Hindu practice. A simple meaning is weaving and expanding energy.

It is slow and is meant to increase intimacy and create a connection with the mind and body that could give powerful orgasms.

Tantric sex or Tantra can be done by anybody that is interested in turning up their sex life and going to new depths with their lovemaking. You might be intrigued by Tanta, but you feel too overwhelmed to explore it. You might have tried it but feel like you need to push your boundaries further and thus taking the practice to another level.

This might sound confusing but if you look at it like this: If a quickie is a takeaway, then tantric sex is a five-star meal that has been lovingly prepared and is worth the wait.

If you can take the effort and time for sex, you will get to a more intense and higher form of ecstasy. Tantra is about understanding and mastering your energy instead of the act. Sexual energy is human nature. Tantra accepts the human nature for itself and elevates it. It doesn't deny or avoid the human desires and nature. Sex is not impure to Tantra. The body is looked at a vessel for enlightenment.

The balance that is created by tantric sex will allow you to be fulfilled. It doesn't chase or deny you the passions and pleasures of life.

Conventional Tantra instructors focus on just the idea of sexuality. This is separate from the original teachings. Most Neo-Tantra workshops are sex education workshops.

Tantra wasn't originally meant to improve relationships or a way to have better sex. It was not practiced by couples. It helped individuals reach a higher level of consciousness. It allowed them the experience of entering nirvana. Some Tantric sects embrace sexual activity. These practices are designed to give the practitioner orgasmic intensity as a way to divine energy. It was never meant to be about enjoying sex. It is spiritual training.

Different models of Tanta or as some call it sacred sexuality have risen and will provide some benefits to couples and individuals. The practice of Tantra can benefit everybody especially couples since it transforms the individual. Couples can find balance, fulfillment, and harmony instead of expecting or demanding it from your partner. This path will lead to depression, resentment, guilt, and the dissolution of the domestic partnership.

Tantra gives the couple a way they can approach the relationship as sacred out and in the bedroom. By bringing their attention consciously to their shared times together, they will be keeping their love alive.

Sex has a great potential for intense pleasure when both partners are mindful and aware. The senses wake up when the heart is open.

Celebrities like Sting and Tom Hanks have commented on how great tantric sex is. Sting's wife Trudie Styler has boasted that Sting can make love for over five hours without stopping.

Tantric sex would be right for you if:

- You are looking to find new things to do in bed.

- You want to be more intimate with your significant other

- You want to reconnect with your partner.

Tantric sex is not goal oriented. This means that you don't have to work too hard to learn it.

The main thing is not to worry about the orgasm but focus on the foreplay being more rewarding and enjoyable until you want to take it to the end.

This can be easier said than done. To delay orgasm, experts use massage, breathing control, and meditation.

If you want to try it do the following:

- Begin by turning down the lights and shut out the world around you.

- Loosen the body. Tantra is moving energy through your body. Shake your arms and legs vigorously to get energy flowing through your system before you begin.

- Get off the bed. This triggers sleep. You will settle for a quick romp instead of the deep connection and more loving sex that is what Tantra is about.

- Be comfortable. Lay down on the floor with your partner. Slowly begin to touch each other. Take your time to touch every part of the body.

- Experiment. Try different touches like gentle stroking, feathery touches, and firm massage. You want to heighten each other's senses slowly and intensely, so you are building each other to the peak by not completely getting them there. Doing this the right way can make sex longer and keep pleasure going for hours.

- Concentrate on breathing. If your mind begins to wander, focus on breathing. Inhale when your partner exhales. This can help to improve the connection you have with each other and keeps your mind in the present moment.

- Never give up. If you don't last longer than ten minutes, give it another try. Tantra takes the time to figure it out since we are all used to sex the traditional way. We think that sex has a start, middle and ending.

It will take practice, but you can learn to let go of the traditional idea of sex and learn to enjoy sex without concentrating on the conclusion. You will learn to control your body, so you will be able to delay climax and increase how strong your orgasms are.

# History of Tantra

Tantra has many teachings and meanings. You can't think about Tantra as a single practice, path, teaching, or philosophy without others disagreeing with you. The word Tantra refers to something meaningful and coherent. To get a hold on what Tantra is let's take a look at how it got its start.

Tantra is an ancient tradition of techniques, rituals, and principles that are used for cultivating a conscious life in and out of the bedroom. The bedroom is what we usually focus on in the west. Tantra has its roots in many spiritual traditions like Taoism, Buddhism, and Hinduism. These are also the birthplace of Yoga. Tantra's history goes back about 7,000 years. This is longer than any religion that is popular today. For as long as we humans have wondered about our existence, we have stood in awe of the power of our sexual nature and wanted to understand it.

Tantra is unique. Its spiritual practices honor life force and sexual energies. Tantra honors the union of female and male energies.

It could be a woman and man or uniting the feminine and masculine energies in ourselves as a path to oneness.

It is a place where we don't feel alone or separate and can be defined as Bliss or the meeting of the Infinite Love and the Divine. This is where spirit, love, and sex becomes one. We have to surrender our hearts ego. It does take practice, courage, and understanding.

Tantra is a tradition that focuses on the connection between higher consciousness, sexuality, and health. It has a long history.

Tantra yoga is a sexual path. It is a system of practical techniques and rituals that use the creative energy in our mind-body system to propel one into a higher state of consciousness. This energy has the capacity for two individuals to mate and make another life form. It is the original form of nuclear fusion.

To understand this, you have to understand the word sutra. Tantra started being used when Jainism, Buddhism, and other Vedic traditions that are now called Hinduism were dominant in India. The core of all these religions were sutras or key texts. The most famous is the *Kama Sutra*, which is a book about erotic arts and love and is unrelated to any Tantra. The *Sutra of Patanjali* is used by yogis today. Sutra has a meaning of thread. That means that a sutra is a thread of thought or a line of thinking. Some think that sutra referred to the thread that bound the palm leaves together.

If sutra is a single thread of thinking, then a Tantra is the complete system of thought. The meaning of Sanskrit is loom. Not the cloth but the entire machine that the cloth is made on.

Sutras were originally books. Tantras were the teachings that were transmitted from the teacher to the student. Being a largely literate society, books began appearing everywhere. Reference manuals, guidebooks, basically cliff notes of the original teachings. These booklets were called Tantras. Sutras came to mean canonical scriptures that were the heart of the religion. Tantras were summaries of these teachings.

There wasn't anything common in the content of the teachings.

Let's look at the sixth century. The Roman Empire had completely disintegrated. The thought of prosperity and stability inspired each warlord. Illiteracy and ignorance reigned. In India, they were having a time of cultural wealth, renewal, and intellectual advancement. The most vibrant practice that swept over the subcontinent in the Kashmir valley. This was a cultural melting pot. It had ancient religious traditions that worshiped Sakti and Siva. Siva was the essence of consciousness. Sakti was the essence of power. Using the loom metaphor, the weaving of Sakti and Siva with the threads of the Vedic culture along with Jainism and Buddhism that was thriving at this time.

When weaving Sakti and Siva together, some facets are very important. These were oral traditions, so transmission involved a student-teacher relationship. These religions were derived from a matriarchal, shamanic society in the Dravidian cultural. The female was the heart of teaching. Women were usually the most powerful and influential teachers. These traditions gave a powerful ritual and ceremony to mark the point of transition in the practitioner's growth. These were not separated from their everyday lives. There were not monastic tradition or priestly class.

The teachings that started to spread in India had an attraction to the population that was well off or was strong middle class.

This middle class was left out of the caste-conscious religions that originated with the Vedic and the male Buddhism. Unlike the more established and scholarly traditions, the teachings were taught that enlightenment was available immediately. No reincarnation was needed. The divine wasn't seen as a distant or abstract deity or many deities, but an all omnipresent presence that every one of use isn't just a part of but the whole of. The Buddhist concept of nothingness was reinterpreted as an omnipresent consciousness. The physical world was an illusion but not as a deception. Every one of us and the world around us is different projections of consciousness. When we expand into the awareness of the universe, we comprehend the illusion of our otherness, from the divine, the world around us, and each other.

These teachings that continued through the classical era were known as Tantra. Thousands of individual and independent teachers solidified into core heritages with diversity but more commonality.

Kashmir Shaivism was just another religion in India over the next hundreds of years. Tantra extended to what we call Hinduism and most of Buddhism with special survival in the Vajrayana Buddhism in the Himalayas. Tantra was viewed as a spiritual practice that was independent of any religion but was adaptable to all.

The similarities that define Tantra includes the direct relationship between the student and teacher, embodying mindfulness, doing rituals as a way to deepen awareness, rejecting the cultural and religious rules, accepting all people, no matter their gender, language, nationality, etc., direct access to the divine, a belief in the sensual experiences of the body as a part of the divine and not as a distraction from the divine.

There have been some debates on the importance of sexuality in the teachings of mindfulness in the rituals of classical Tantra. It is present. One booklet teaches about the discovery of uniting with the divine through orgasm. One influential teacher was branded and imprisoned for corrupting the Brahmin class in his town with his rituals.

The writings that have survived are profoundly and deeply philosophical teachings from very educated Brahmin class scholars that adopted the practice. These thinkers honored their traditions by keeping their secrets. Just like the cults in ancient Greece, we can only surmise what happened behind closed veils.

The architecture and art are not inconclusive.

The architecture of Vajrayana Buddhism temple, are vivid with imagery of the penis, the vagina and vulva, and deities locked in carnal embraces. Illustrations show the practitioner and consort in sexual unions. It is usually assumed that the man is the practitioner and female are consort, but this is a large misunderstanding. Women and men are equal practitioners when it comes to Tantra. The great teachers were usually female. The great writers were usually male. Classic Tantra died out around the 1100's. Islam came to India and Buddhism went away. The tantric practice began to disappear. It survived in three ways in

Hatha Yoga, the Brahmanic Sri Vidya in southern India, and Vajrayana Buddhism in the Himalayas. Vajrayana Buddhism didn't carry all the aspects of Tantra but preserved many philosophical teachings, rituals, and key texts within the Buddhist context. Sri Vidya was cleaned of many rule-rejecting aspects of Tantra but kept the ritual and philosophy within the Vedic context. Hatha Yoga kept the practices and teaching that embodied mindfulness but without the philosophical depth within the ritual elements.

About 900 years later, Tantra sprang back to life with the ferment, vibrancy, and diversity of its early years. You might be wondering how this could happen.

European spirituality had a tradition of sacred mysticism and sexuality before connecting to the spiritual traditions of Japan, Mongolia, China, Nepal, Tibet, and India. It was this meeting of the minds that Tantra came back to life. Inspired by the teachings of the Tantra texts, western sexuality reformulated its thinking and reconstituted itself. It incorporated the understanding of breathing, mindfulness, and energy with the spirituality of the divine.

Tantra was born again.

Some teachers and schools align themselves with the teaching of traditional Tantra. Others are teaching forms of Vajrayana that have been adapted and simplified for the Western lifestyle. Yoga teachers have discovered the sexual dimensions within their craft and have reconstructed the Tantra that gave birth to it.

Since its transition in the 1970s to the west, it has been practiced in several different ways. It all depends on the teacher.

There are four types of Tantra:

White Tantra is a purely esoteric practice that works with sex as energy through meditation that uses visualization and breath. It seeks the divine through enlightenment. It is practiced individually.

Red Tantra uses white tantric practices and works with the body using sexual techniques with a partner.

Pink Tantra is what is commonly practiced in the west. It uses both red and white practices and focuses on devotional practices and a couple's relationship to bring sexual energy through the heart.

Black Tantra uses sexual energy to manifest changes outside the practitioner, in the environment, in others and is not used much now.

Tantra has nothing to do with religion. You can find a lot of its practices and symbols all throughout history, and from many different religions and cultures. As far back as 2000 BC in the old Egyptian kingdom, and the Indus Valley, you can see the representation of the non-duality of the inner marriage and the way it represents the binding of the feminine and masculine principles. The principles of Tantra are deeply rooted in religions such as Christianity, Sufism, and Judaism. You can find another strand of Tantra in Taoism.

During the years of 300 and 400 CE, in India, Tantra began to emerge when the Buddhists and the Hindus wrote the first Tantric texts. These writings were poetic metaphors that pointed to Divine love and oneness. They wrote them is such a way that only the ones that wrote them could understand them. Tantric teachings were guarded closely and were given to the disciple from the master orally after they had gone through purification and preparation.

Tantra began to peak around the 11th and 12th centuries. It was a widely and openly practiced thing in India. Tantra spoke out against the belief that a person could only be liberated by renouncing the world and rigorous asceticism. The yogis who taught Tantra thought that human suffering was caused from the notion of separation. Tantra advocated celebrating the sensual, and when you do so, you find the transcendence of the physical

Tantra is practiced in three different forms: the wandering yogis, the monastic tradition, and the householder tradition. Hinduism has many laws and rules, including a class division. Tantra has always been non-denominational, and anyone is able to practice it within his or her daily lives.

Meditations for weaving were used by weavers as they thought about the undifferentiated and interwoven existence of nature. Meditations on drinking, lovemaking, and eating was practice by queens and kings.

When India was invaded in the 13th century, the Tantrics were slaughtered, and their manuscripts were destroyed. Tantra went underground and had remained there since. The Tibetan monasteries preserved Tantric Buddhism. When the Chinese invaded Tibet, nuns and monks were murdered, and their manuscripts were destroyed. The ones who escaped found ways to spread their knowledge.

The Tantric paths are divided into two groups. One group is where an individual practitioner will work on their sexual energy, and they are referred to as White Tantra. The Tantric groups that include contact with a partner are referred to as Red Tantra. These are more prominent in the modern system.

In the western world, you can find practices in the Tibetan Buddhist tradition, and you can be taught in the Kriya and Kundalini yoga schools. These are White Tantra. The Taoist tradition, with a slight change, is a Red Tantra path.

Daniel Odier mainly teaches the tandava or the sitting meditation. In this form of mediation, the practitioners try to become more connected with refined states of divine tremoring that helps them to connect with the Kashmiri energy massage and the essence of life.

The Tantric practices and texts involve a large range of topics mostly spiritual and not sexual. Tantrism is known in the West is known anti-morality elements. It is stereotypically portrayed as something that preachers sex and eroticism in the name of religion. One that is loaded with alcohol and offering meat to deities. Jayanta Bhatta, a 9th-century scholar, stated that Tantric practices and ideas are perfecting, but there are immoral teachings like in the Nilambara sect. Their practitioners wear a blue garment and engage in uncontrolled public sex at festivals. Bhatta wrote that this was not necessary and threatened the values of society.

Sexuality has been a large part of Tantra. Sexual fluids have been looked upon as substances of power and have been used ritualistically. Some practices are extreme and exceptional. They aren't found in many of the Hindu or Buddhist practices and literature. There are some texts where scholars tend to disagree, such as the Kaula tradition where they view sexual fluids as a power substance and is mentioned ritually.

In most Buddhist and Hindu Tantra texts, the extreme forms of sexual rituals are absent. In Jain, tantric text, it is absent. But sex, eroticism, and emotions are regarded in Tantric literature as desirable, natural, and a way to transform the deity within us. It is to recapitulate and reflect the bliss of Shakti and Shiva. Kama or sex is an aspect of life and the root of the universe. Kama's purpose goes beyond procreation and is a means to spiritual fulfillment.

# Benefits

Tantra is more than just enhancing one's lovemaking skills. It can teach us to be aware of the life force that flows through us and how to guide the flow consciously. The more you can flow with it, the more it will flow to and through you to energize your life. The energy flowing through your brain and body is rejuvenating, balancing, and nourishing. Couples that practice Tantra together can give each other the gift of life through joy and pleasure. This is the greatest gift we can give each other. It is priceless.

By creating a harmonious union of the female and male aspects in each of us, Tantra can help us understand how these forces can heal and enlighten each other.

This results in a heightened state of awareness. It gives us access to great energy that can be channeled into full body orgasms. This is mind expanding, energizing, exhilarating, and exciting. It gives us knowledge of our essence or the force that created us so that we can live with our radiant and most beautiful self.

Tantra teaches how to achieve this awareness in our lives and how we can apply this force to each aspect of our lives.

Many find that Tantra increases their alertness, provides a deep calmness, enhanced well-being, and greater vitality. Some might even begin to feel smarter and excel in their chosen profession.

The benefits can be felt emotionally, physically, spiritually and creatively.

Researchers are discovering what Tantrics have known for years: a fulfilling emotional and sexual life is beneficial to our state of mind and overall health.

Stronger orgasms can boost the immune system. It can even stimulate hormones that increase people's physical and emotional well-being and strengthen the heart and other organs.

With Tantric practices, women and men gain a better understanding of the deeper states of orgasm. They could come together in multiple times. A man might experience an orgasm without feeling depleted as with normal sex.

This orgasmic state can lead to feeling more energetic, passionate, and alive in every area of our lives. Feeling energized, nurtured, and loved is the best cure for depression and many other ailments.

The benefits of practicing Tantric Sex are many. Tantric sexual states have been associated with similar states that are achieved with meditation. The purpose of these sexual energy states to become one with as person's life consciousness. Sexual activity has positive benefits for the psyche and the body.

When the body reaches a high state of arousal, the body will release hormones that will create a euphoric sense that will flood into the endocrine system. Sexual energy has the ability to nourish the human body and provides with a sense of being alive.

When a person makes love, they are opening up their hearts to another person and giving their self the chance to give and receive pleasure.

Sacred sexuality takes us past all this to teach us of the deeper realms of the human psyche and gives us the true compassion and understanding. With sensual and passionate awareness you are able to increase the quality of sex life.

By practicing Tantric Sex, you will get the opportunity to awaken your Kundalini energy. This is great for you. Through Tantric sex, you will begin to understand your sexual energy power. One of the most powerful energies in the world is sexual energy. When you cultivate this energy, it can bring about an ecstatic state of being. This can help to you heal you emotionally and physically. When in an orgasmic state for an extended period of time, you are able to process through an emotional state easier and receive pleasure at the same time. This is one way to have fun while clearing out emotional energy. Tantra involves self-realization, intimacy, and honest communication.

Self-realization is infinite and goes beyond time and space. This leads to complete unity consciousness, contentment, and peace of mind. There is no need to change spiritual beliefs either. Tantra might also include accessing high states of consciousness as the main objective. For many practitioners, it offers a way to enhance, expand, and enrich their lovemaking. You first begin with sex, then love, then prayer, then transcendence. So, we move from the gross to the subtle. In transcendence, sex, love, and prayer all have to completely disappear. Make it peaceful, silent, meditative where not a trace is left. These four stages make us use the traditional yoga meditation, breathing, and positions. This is taught outside of the Hindu religion and culture. A unique aspect of Tantra is the New Age belief of include massage, counseling, and Reichian bodywork.

Here are some reasons to develop a Tantric sex practice:

1. Deeper Connection: Couples who explore a Tantric practice report feelings of closeness and being able to overcome problems better than they used to. Awareness of your partner, syncing of breaths, and eye contact can help to bring your relationship to another level.

2. Patience: The Art of Tantra is slow moving. Yes, this means that awkward moments will abound. This is why many of us only have sex in a dark room with our eyes closed. Being able to work through the confusing positions, the meditation of holding back an orgasm, and the connection you feel with your partner will develop the skill of learning to be patient.

3. Problem Solving: The Kama Sutra positions aren't easy to get into for beginners. Learning how to prolong the experience without orgasming can require changing positions and trial and error. The need to work and talk together in these vulnerable moments can expand our problem-solving skills.

4.  Creativity: We benefit from embracing supra-sexuality by expressing one's life purpose, empowerment, and creativity to emancipate or potential. Sex is used to create human life, but it can be used to create life projects by bringing energy and attention to your goals while having sex.

5.  Selflessness: During Tantra, you will benefit from holding back your orgasm. Beyond pleasure and procreation, Tantric Sex has the power to liberate. This is an ecstatic experience that is compared to getting a glimpse into our cosmic consciousness. Don't worry if you don't get there the first time you try, especially if your partner is drifting past you. If you can support each other's out-of-orgasm launch into the heavens can help us to remember that giving is better than receiving.

6.  Empowerment. Do not confuse this with power. We have been doing this for far too long. An organic, authentic sexual practice could help us get back to being humble by stripping away our egos and pretenses. Empowerment comes after all that. Feeling as if you don't have anything to be ashamed of, or hide, can bring a wonderful sense of purpose. It gives the ability to express or greatest loves and deepest fears. There will be no more hiding under sheets.

## Sexual Secrets

Stay in the Current Moment: A lot of people tend to miss out on the things around them because they don't know how to be at the moment. Be present so that you won't miss any of the fun.

Make the conditions right. Turn off any distractions, focus, take advantage of your desires and feel rested.

Cultivate sexual mindfulness. Allow yourself to be attentive, erotic, and playful. Allow yourself to become involved in this sensory moment.

Make an exciting atmosphere. Use music, the magic of incense, the scents of aromatherapy, and the power of light.

Entice yourself using natural aphrodisiacs. You can find many aphrodisiacs in nature such as coco, fruits, and oysters.

Allow your mind to open. If you keep expectations, you run the risk of ruining the moment. Keep mind things that will bring back your youthful energy, empowerment, and enlightenment.

Let all your fears go. Your inhibitions are worthless and will block who your dream to be. You should be completing yourself. When you can allow yourself to release fears, the more you will become aroused, and the more this will impact your sexual experiences.

Notice your surroundings. Notice every sensation, emotion, sound, environment, and breathing. It doesn't matter if you are with a partner or alone.

Notice the power of colors. You can use color therapy by using different lingerie, fabrics, candles, or lighting so you can bring more color into your surroundings.

Tap into your chakra energy. Your chakras are energy points along your central axis. Each point has an energy that can be expressed in certain emotions, attitudes, and actions.

Charge your Kundalini. This is a life force energy that originated in India that will awaken a student and merge the spiritual natures.

Lose control. Allow you and your partner to take turns leading. Allow yourself to give up power has the possibility to be arousing

Flow with the rhythm. Let yourself to become entrained. This is when two moving bodies lock into one another so that they are able to vibrate in harmony

Take your time. We will only find the road to complete fulfillment by allowing yourself to explore all of your erotic landscapes and by allowing yourself to savor your body's hot spots.

Express your joy. If you like what you are feeling, tell your partner. When you're vocal, it can help to entice your partner. If they don't like it, try showing them where they should touch.

Make the choice of release or not. It doesn't matter if you believe in the release of energy or transmitting the sexual energy throughout different channels, you have to make sure that there is pleasure in a sacred union.

Reach new heights. Find the deep relationships between spirituality and sexuality.

The important thing is sex. Sex is able to heal your energy in your body, spirit, and mind.

Honor this pleasure as a gift. This is an honest aspect using the creative life force that electrifies every part of your life.

Create pure ecstasy. The purpose of this is to create high arousal states while you are also relaxed.

For most of us, sex is the most spiritual experience. Unfortunately, our culture doesn't view sex this way. Sex is degraded and debased as no more than a primal nuisance that we haven't outgrown. This magical, potent practice can give life, not just to each other, but to a deeper communion and understanding with an etheric, elusive world, if we are brave enough to go beyond the end goal of orgasm.

# Tantric Positions

If you are inspired by the success of the ancient teachings, here is a list of tantric positions to tease, tempt and thoroughly, please. Grab your partner and a take a trip toward erotic enlightenment.

## The Mermaid

Lie face up on the end of a desk, countertop, or bed. Put a pillow beneath your buttocks to create a bit of elevation. Keep your legs extended up in the air with them together. If you need to, you can place your hands underneath your pillow to help elevate your hips. Your partner will then enter you from a standing position. If what you're laying on is lower, then he can kneel. He can use your feet for leverage. This will also help to give him some extra stability so that he is able to thrust deeply.

This one you will love. If you keep your leg together, this will make him feel bigger inside you. You will be creating a lot of friction and a wonderfully tight fit for him. Drive yourself wild and show off for him by self-stimulating your clitoris as he is thrusting.

## The Sofa Spread-Eagle

Stand on the edge of a couch, bed, or if you have incredible balance, two chairs with your legs opened wide. Your partner will be standing in front of you. Bend your knees to adjust your stance if needed so he can slide between them and get to your center. Rock your bodies to create bliss.

There is nothing is nothing better than the need it now, impulsive sex while standing. This position spares you the pain of trying to match up the private parts. While this stance will allow you to move with his rhythm, your spread legs will give you a vulnerable, super-sexy feeling. All the frontal friction will hit your clitoris and take you to a no hands needed climax.

## Torrid Tidal Wave

This one is great for a secluded beach. There is no other pose when you are interested in taking a make out session to a passionate plateau. Your partner will be at the edge of the water on his back. His legs should be straight and together. You will then straddle his penis, and stretch over him so that you are lying with your pelvises aligned. Lift up your chest, and let your hands hold your weight. You create the speed on this one as you rock with the waves.

With each pull and push, your clitoris will rub along his pelvic bone creating toe curling friction. Every move will send sensations boosting currents through every nerve of your body. Now and then clench your butt cheeks tight so you can feel his throbbing penis inside you.

## Tub Tangle

Have you partner relining in a filled tub, straddle him, and face him. When you have him inside you, he will sit up so that you are both facing each other. You should both now wrap your legs around each other, and then hook your elbows under each other's knees, and lift them to chest level. Hold each other tightly as you move into ecstasy.

This is a perfect position for a confined space because it allows you to twine your bodies around each other, which makes a cozy connection that is perfect for intimacy. Since your mouths are nearby, indulge in passionate kissing. Don't forget to nibble on the neck and ears.

## Lap Dance

You will need a chair with a tall back. Pad it with a pillow and have him sit down. Straddle his hardness and lean back just a bit. Put your hands on his knees. Raise your legs, one at a time, until each ankle is resting on his shoulders. Pump you rear at a speed that will make you both moan. To give you more power, balance all of your weight between your hands and ankles.

This position has great intimacy potential. This gets you extremely close. This erotic view will give your man lasting memories for weeks. Spice it up with some lingerie that you can seductively take off and toss to him that will add more steam to the session.

## The G-Force

While lying on your back, bring your knees into your chest. Your partner should kneel in front. He can grab hold of your feet if he wants. This is the angle he will penetrate you from. If you want to add more awesome action, place your feet on his chest, and he grabs hold of your hips. This will give him more control, allowing for deeper penetration.

You will be giving him the reins for this one, but it will be worth it. For the ones who know how powerful the G-spot is, this deep, intense penetration will have you moaning in no time. There is no excuse for him not doing double duty. This position is perfect for him to be inside you while stimulating your clitoris with his hand.

## Rock a Bye Booty

With your partner lying down, slowly straddle him. Once he is inside, have him sit up so that you are facing each other. Now wrap your legs behind each other's buttocks. Hook your elbows under the other person's knees. Cradle each other.

This will limit how much you can thrust; you both will still receive pleasure if you sway back and forth. Start slowly and allow your rhythm to increase. As you momentum increase, squeeze your pelvic muscles to keep him hard. Yes, these are the same muscles you contract when you are trying not to urinate on yourself. This tightens your grip on his penis while moving blood to your private parts and increase your enjoyment.

Since you are both close, this is a great position to become more intimate. In fact, this opens up a lot of options for kissing. Kissing each other's necks or sucking on earlobes will bring you closer.

## Baby Got Back

Your partner will kneel and sit on his heels. Stand with your back to him then lower onto his penis by squatting or doing a plie with your feet placed on either side of his legs. Tease him; then go deeper until you are resting on his lap. Your thighs and butt curves into him.

This is a chick in charge position. There is nothing like him begging for you to go just an inch or two more. His whimpering will be your delight. He has a great rear view and receives pleasure with each long, super orgasmic stroke when you begin to pump up and down.

To get maximum pleasure, position yourself in front of a mirror and watch yourself. Watching a sexy session makes it even hotter.

## The Passion Pretzel

Kneel facing each other. Each one will put the opposite foot flat on the ground and scoot closer until your genital join up. Lean forward on your feet; for a slow romp you will lunge back and forth.

This puts you both in the same stance and sharing the reins while you rock each other's world. Since you aren't using your arms, think about the different places you can touch. There might not be a lot of in and out action, your grinding will provide great clitoral contact and will allow for the gradual ascent to that climactic cloud nine.

## The Amazing Butterfly

The key here is getting lined up correctly with your partner. Find a place where you can lie down, and he will stand in front of you. There is a catch. It needs to be somewhere that will put your pelvis a foot lower than his. Raise your legs up to his shoulders and rest them there. Tilt up your pelvis so that the back forms a straight line that angles towards him. Once the privates are angled together, he will hold your butt at the best angle.

This position is great for amazing ecstasy without any need for a lot of energy commitment. The tilt of the pelvis will give the penis the best access to the vagina and will build more friction for both involved. When this is done slowly, it is dreamlike. This orgasm will make you feel as if you are flying

To add more pleasure, use some solo action. Use the hand that's free to stimuli your clitoris. When he notices that you are bringing on your own bliss, it will send his desire soaring.

## Get Down on It

The partner needs to get in the lotus position with both of his legs crossed and the heels place on top of his knees. Face him, sit in your partner's lap and mount him with your legs positioned around his waist. Embrace each other and kiss with a shared breath. When you exhale, your guy will inhale. As you do this breathing, rock your pelvis back and tighten your vaginal muscles. When you exhale, rock forward and release your vaginal muscles. Your guy will mirror your movements.

This position is perfect for yoga fanatics. Syncing your breathing and moving at the same time will help to increase your intimacy as you ride the waves to an amazing climax.

Take it slowly getting into this position. Relaxing is the key. Add music and candles to help set the mood. Loosen each other up with massages. To enhance the massage using aromatic oils, make sure you are both slicked down.

## Row His Boat

Your partner will slouch in a comfortable chair with their legs spread out slightly. Facing him, straddle his lap with knees open and bent over the chair. You will brace your feet against the seat. As he is holding your butt, hips, or thighs, you will hold onto the back of the chair and start moving up and down.

This is a traditional girl on top with a tantalizing twist. By having your knees bent and your hands and feet using the chair as a springboard, it becomes a bouncy position. It's perfect if you want to tease your partner with your movements. Switch things up by moving in circle shapes. You are both close enough for kissing, touching, or giving looks.

## The Wow Him Powwow

Have your partner sit down with his legs crossed. Face him and straddle his legs. Lower yourself onto his lap. DO NOT penetrate yet. Wrap your legs around each other, so they are hugging his butt. Then, as you are holding each other tightly, he will enter you. Begin to rock back and forth slowly, increase your speed as you get closer to climax.

Just like the standard missionary position, this one takes closeness and eye contact to the next level. This comfortable position encourages equal control over the timing and speed of the thrusts. This allows for the gradual buildup of pleasure for each partner. Your clitoris is at a great angle, too. This will allow him to stroke you without interrupting the action.

## The Hot Seat

Have your partner kneel behind you, but make sure he leans slightly backward. Keeping your back toward him, you kneel in front of him. Your legs will be between his. You both will be squeezed together. He will wrap his arms around your waist. He can put his hands wherever he wants. When he is inside, move in circular movements or up and down. Stop to take breaks if you need to.

With his tilted position, he has perfect access to the G-spot. You will also have extra pressure in this position because you're pushing your butt into his groin.

## Yab Yum

Your partner will sit on the floor in the lotus position. He will help you into his lap. When you are completely penetrated, wrap your legs around his back. The position of your partner's penis could penetrate the cervix and thus allow you to achieve a cervical-uterine orgasm. You have the active role in this position.

You will then need to move your pelvis back and forth while your vaginal muscles are contracted. This position allows you to be penetrated extremely deeply.

This posture allows you to meditate together. This allows meditation to be part of your intercourse. Thus, making it part of the spiritual ascent and gives you to get to a simultaneous orgasm. Keeping eye contact and feeling your partner's body is key in tantric sex, so this position is perfect. His hands are free, so they can stimulate and roam all over your body. You are aligned to share lots of passionate kisses.

## The Sidewinder

This position is face to face also that allows for kissing and eye contact. This one uses the spooning position by with both partners facing each other. It is relatively easy getting into this position. Start off in the missionary position and then roll onto your side. Use what's comfortable for you. You may keep one leg under him, or both can be together resting across his legs. Focus on breathing together and get in tune with the other's movements.

## The Padlock

Get up on the washing machine or counter top and wrap your legs around your partner's waist. He will have control of this position. He can grab onto your butt or hips. Lean back and rest on your elbows or hands to create some distance. Enjoy the view of your bodies joined.

## The Double Decker

This is one of the greatest positions for mutual satisfaction. Start by sitting in reverse cowgirl and then lay back against his chest. Take control by putting your feet on the bed to help you slide up and down on his hardness. Enjoy his warm breath on your neck and be aware of his cues to either speed up or slow down.

## Time Bomb

Get a chair and have him sit. Lower yourself on him until your feet can touch the floor and you have reached full penetration. You are in the driver's seat; your partner can grab your hips and guide your motions. Slow down or speed up and help each other reach that simultaneous orgasm.

## The Ascent to Desire

This is an athletic sex position. Your partner will sit on the bed, and you will sit down on him while facing him. Put your legs on his back. Hold onto his neck for support. Once you are completely penetrated, he will stand up while supporting your butt with his arms. You can leave your legs around his back or put the on the bed for more balance. You can lean back slightly and work your hips. This one might not be for every couple, but it is extremely exciting if you dare to try.

Practicing this requires physical stability from your partner since he needs to be able to support your and engage in intercourse at the same time.

## The Bow

Lay down on your back; your partner will lift your pelvis. He will sit between your calves. Cross your legs and put them on his chest and then he will penetrate you. He will support himself with his knees and fingertips on the ground. He can move passionately at a firm and slow pace. The penetration will be deep. The vagina will decrease in size in this position. This position allows the man to reach your cervix. You just might reach a cervical-uterine orgasm. Only a few women ever experience this type of orgasm.

This posture amplifies the vital and sexual energy and is felt at both the beginning of sex and at the end when both of you feel the need of being invigorated by the vital force.

## The Great Bee

Help your partner lie down on his back on the bed or floor. Sit on top of him in a squatting position on his thighs. Firmly tighten your calves after you have completely penetrated yourself with his penis. Support yourself by placing your hands on your partner's chest. Begin riding his hardness by pushing yourself up and down. Change the pace by going in a circular pattern. Rotate your hips as wide as possible.

If you feel that the pleasure is reaching the climax too quickly, stop and focus on your breathing along with your partner. Your movements need to be kept under control and be in agreement with your partner's control and energy.

## The Embraced Posture

This needs to be done on a surface where your pelvises will line up. Lie on your back with your legs crossed and up in the air. Your partner will penetrate you carefully and passionately. The position of your legs helps to control the vaginal muscles and help you move to that your pelvises stay aligned. For your partner, this posture is great if you can do vaginal muscle contractions.

Your partner needs to be careful and able to control his energy. The intense pleasure will make it difficult to maintain sexual continence. You might feel some empathy for you partner. You can adjust your movements to help him control keeping the climax at bay.

## Doggie Style

A lot of couples prefer positions where the man penetrates from behind. The normal on is where you will kneel on all fours, and your partner will penetrate you from behind. This position is excellent for deep penetration and the stimulation of the G-spot.

Your partner will be impressed by your movements. He can reach around and under to massage your breasts or clitoris. The movements can be many from the back and forth, to circular, slow to deep pounding to excite both of you.

## The Pressed Posture

You will lie on your back and slowly raise your legs and put them on your partner's chest. The feeling of your feet on his chest is extremely enjoyable and creates intimacy. This posture creates a wonderful compression that will lead to you contracting your vaginal muscles and decreases the vagina's size. Your partner will penetrate you as normal. This position allows pleasurable sensations that are felt by both of you leading to achieve a prolonged orgasm.

## Half Pressed Posture

You will lie down on your back and slowly raise your legs. Stretch one leg out straight and place the other on your partner's chest. Your partner will penetrate you as normal. In this posture, you have more freedom of movement so you can alternate your legs. Stretching out the right one and bending the left then stretching the left and bending the right. This position will allow the same pleasurable sensations that can be felt by both and leads to a prolonged orgasm.

## Tiger Walk

You lean forward on your arms and knees. Sit with your butt raised and your head down. Your partner will kneel behind your, holding your waist. Slowly he will penetrate you. A secret from the Taoist teachings says that it is important for the penis to penetrate as deeply as possible. Then alternate each five superficial movements with eight deep strokes. While holding his ejaculation back, your partner has to continue until your vagina expands and contracts spontaneously and releases the essence of Yin abundantly. Both need to relax deeply and be aware of the impact of this posture for at least 45 minutes.

## Turned Dragon

The happiness of being a human who loves is the pleasure and joy of the other human that lets themselves be loved and loves without asking for anything in return. If your partner can do this position without ejaculating will make your experience completely fulfilling. Your partner will gain a state of flourishing health because a hundred sufferings have disappeared.

You will lie on your back while your partner lies on top of you. He will support himself on his knees. Lift your pelvis as he slowly enters you. He has the freedom of massaging your breasts, arms, and shoulders. Your partner will move rhythmically and slowly, alternating two deep movements with eight superficial ones. The movement will be made by your partner with force and strength. Continuously controlling his ejaculation. His penis goes into your vagina while semi-erect and is removed when still hard.

## The Butterfly Elan

Your partner will sit in an armchair with his legs spread slightly apart. You will sit on top of his hugging his thighs while facing him. Your feet will rest against the chair. You are in charge. Move slowly at first then switch to faster movements leaning on his arms. Your partner can play with your clitoris, breast, or whatever he can reach.

## The Ape

You will spread your legs slightly, lean forward, and place your palms on the floor or chair. Your partner will stand behind you and holds your waist with his hands. He will slowly enter you and penetrate with deep strokes. Bring her multiple times to the verge of orgasm without ejaculating. Your partner has the freedom to massage your breast, clitoris or whatever he can reach. He can hold your thighs and gets a deeper penetration and a wonderful stimulation of the G-spot. Both of you will be surrounded with energy waves crossing your bodies from top to bottom, experiencing wonderful pleasure.

## The Elephant

You will lie on your side offering your partner a wonderful view of your vagina and arched back. If you are lying on your left side, keep the left leg straight and bend the right leg at the knee. Your partner gets between your legs so to speak with his right leg between your thighs. Your right thigh will be on top of his right leg. He will bend like an elephant with his lower back pushed in he enters your vagina slowly while you encourage him with seductive movements. This allows for easier penetration. He changes positions slightly to get on his knees while keeping control and adjusting the depth and pace of his strokes. He tempers the force, so he doesn't damage your vagina. You will firmly squeeze your vagina around his penis leading him toward a wonderful orgasm.

There are some variations to this pose with you starting in the tiger walk pose, and both of you will descend at the same time into the elephant pose while staying intimately united.

Another variation is you can stretch your right leg or whichever leg is bent over your partner's leg to experiment a deeper range of erotic pleasures.

This position with side penetration is extremely pleasurable for you since it favors deep penetration and stimulates the cervix. This experience can give you a cervical-uterine orgasm. Your partner can be attentive to you by moving your right hip to reach the sensitive places in your vagina. You will be able to concentrate on the pleasure you are experiencing in your cervix. Your partner can caress every inch of your body that he can reach to intensify your orgasms.

## Splitting of a Bamboo

This position resembles the great opening posture. You will lie on your back and raise one leg and place it on your partner's shoulder. Your partner will get on his knees and hug your leg that is on his shoulder. Your other leg will remain on the bed. While your partner makes love to you, you will alternate moving your legs from shoulder to bed.

Your partner will touch, with wavy movements of his hips, new depths of pleasure inside your vagina, which embraces her with sweetness. Your partner can look at your fondly while massaging all parts of your body.

## The Erotic Carousel

In the Kama Sutra, it says that it is recommended that the woman takes an active role during lovemaking. The woman should at least once during lovemaking take the initiative. The Kama Sutra shares two way that the woman can have an active role. She is in control from the beginning or at some point during lovemaking; she gets on top without interrupting the action. The erotic texts speak about the role of the woman when she is the initiator for her lover, teaching them the mysteries of controlled pleasure or sexual continence.

This position is a very exciting position. It can arouse intense feelings of passion and generates an explosive orgasm.

Your partner will lie down on his back, and you will sit on top facing away from him. Lean on your feet and hold your spine straight. You will move up and down with sensuality.

This gives you great freedom. You can search for certain penetration angles that work for you, then change your pelvic position to switch to other areas. Inside your vagina are many areas that can arouse certain feelings and you will be able to be fully aware of them and enjoy them in abundance.

This position will bring both of you to enhanced states of passion. They will gradually give your explosive orgasms. You must pay attention to both your state and your partner's state. You can help him control his sexual energy.

## Relaxed Arch

Your partner will need to be on the floor or bed with their legs stretched out. You will crawl close to him on your knees and climb into his lap. When you have fully penetrated yourself on his penis, arch your back slowly but without hurting your lower back. Lean back and put your head on the bed between your partner's legs and hold his ankles with your hands. Your lover's hands will firmly but gently hold your lower back and help your movements. You will be deliciously surprised when your lover bends over you and enjoys the ripeness of your breasts.

For lovers who are eager to taste the sensuality of this posture. Even just a few minutes of making love in this position will be memorable. This allows the stimulation of the anterior wall of the vagina, so all your pleasure points in this area will be aroused. The G-spot is caressed and gratified by the relaxed arch.

## The Anvil

Lie down on your back with your legs in the air. Your partner will kneel down and penetrate you slowly. Next, he will begin leaning over you and push your legs back over your shoulders. This creates a feeling of intense pressure. It will end up with your man right on top with your legs between both or you. In this position, you are completely submissive to him. He sets up the pace for this position from agonizingly slow to deep pounding to drive you both wild.

## Aphrodite

Begin by caressing each other's bodies. When you both are ready for the act, your partner will sit down comfortable stretching his legs out in front of him. You will sit on his lap horizontally. You will get some breast to chest friction with this one. Your partner will lift your thighs and pull you onto his penis. He is in charge of the pace of this one. Set the tempo slow at first and then increase as you feel you need to. With you facing sideways, he has the opportunity of sucking and nibbling on your neck and breasts. With your free hands, you can stimulate both your clitoris and his testicles giving both of you the time of your life.

## Session Tips

Practice these tips to reconnect with your lover. You will soon master that art of Tantra.

Take Time to Have a Weekly Session: Try to commit to a weekly tantric session with your partner. Choose a time and day that works for both. Set aside two hours to celebrate your relationship. Don't reschedule even if you feel tired. Your tantric session will invigorate you and make you feel the stronger energy flowing through you. Stick to your date. Only reschedule if necessary. You will be amazed by the increased playfulness, connection, and love every session will bring to you both.

*Try Something New:* Have fun and don't be so serious. Have an open heart and open mind, even if it sounds silly. Many who are new to tantra have said the eye-gazing is awkward and weird. That is until they tried. Never dismiss anything. Set some practices to the side until you are ready to experiment. Make sure to remain curious and playful. If what you are practicing feels good, you are one step closer.

*Set the Mood:* Prepare by adorning and cleaning the bed with comfy blanket and cushion. Create a sensual place by having candles, flowers, drinks and some eats that you both like. Turn your bedroom into a love temple. Light lots of candles. The dim light will bring magic into space. Put on some relaxing music that will play for two hours. Make sure the temperature in the room so both can be comfortable and relax.

*Take a Relaxing Bath:* Run a bubble bath for your love. Light candles all over the bedroom and music and spread rose petal on the floor. Pour a glass of their favorite beverage. Take it one step further and join them.

*Shake Your Body Alive:* Release any blockages or tension by re-sensitizing your body. Stand to face each other with feet spread hip width apart. Keep your knees slightly bent. Take a minute to relax from head to toe and shake your whole body for five minutes. Be sure to shake your legs, shoulders, head, hips, hands, and arms. You will love the tingling you experience after. This helps your body to experience pleasure in a more intense and deeper way.

*Meditate:* Meditate together to connect your hearts and clear your minds. Sit cross-legged facing each other and close your eyes. Breathe deeply. Just be together in silence until all the worries are gone. This helps you become fully focused and present with each other. You can play a guided meditation, meditative music, or sit silently.

**Tell Your Partner What You Love About Them:** Look them in the eye and start every sentence with "I love...". Be authentic and true, reach deep into your heart and express everything you appreciate about them. This isn't the time for discussion just sharing. Open your hearts deeper and create intimacy and connection, use the following and fill in the blanks with your words. "My heart desires...", "It brings me great pleasure when you...". When you have finished, invite your partner to do the same for you and thank them.

**Look Into Each Other's Eyes:** Look your partner in the eye. The eyes are the gateway to the soul. Ask them to look at you, too. Try to hold the gaze for 5 to 15 minutes. It will feel like such a long time when you begin until you can connect on the soul level. This connection feels delicious and wonderful. To deepen this, synchronize your breaths, so you will inhale and exhale in the same moment.

**Sit in the Yab-Yum Pose:** This pose is great to connect intimately with your partner. Your partner will sit down cross-legged while you sit on top of his legs facing each other. This can be done clothed or naked. Embrace each other and breathe together. Allow your bodies to become tuned to each other. Let them merge in this beautiful embrace. Feel the love your share. The joy of celebrating your relationship. The appreciation for the wonderful moment.

*Engage in a Tantric Kiss:* Continue sitting in the above pose, breath together and think about sharing your breaths. Join your lips in a gentle, soft kiss. Allow the lips the meld together in a sensual kiss. Savor and relax the kiss as you caress your partner's lips with yours. Stay at the moment and immerse yourself in the sensations of intimacy and closeness.

*Give and Receive a Tantric Massage:* Take turns giving and receiving a massage. Have your partner lie face down as you wake up their body to different sensations. Softly touch their skin with fingertips, hot wax, ice, feathers, fabrics, and flowers. Start with a gentle touch, then get fuller, longer strokes. Begin with the non-erogenous zones like the feet, legs, hands, head, neck, and back. Slowly excite their energy by touching their genitals, inner thighs, and butt. Have them turn over and repeat on the front of their body. Awaken their skin with a soft touch, and then massage their non-erogenous zones before moving on to their genitals, inner thighs, nipples, breasts. Ask for feedback and remind them to relax, breathe and stay present. This massage isn't about orgasm, don't try to make them come just enjoy giving them pleasure.

*Take It Slow:* When you are ready to add the physical contact into your practice, go slow. Extremely slow. Start with just holding hands. You can try putting your hand over your partner's heart or sitting in their lap. Continue to hold eye contact or synchronize your breathing while touching. This is a chance to know your partner's body better and set boundaries. Keep the play exploratory.

*Stay In The Moment:* A large part of Tantra is learning to stay grounded and be aware of everything you are feeling. Don't force yourself to feel something else at the moment. The goal is the pleasure, not the orgasm. Separate the sex from the climax is tough but it is possible. We are a culture where the goal is the climax, so if we don't achieve one, then the sex was horrible. You can have great sex without having an orgasm. Keep this in mind when playing with your partner. Avoid touching your partner's genitals and don't let them touch yours. Think about where to touch your partner if you aren't trying to make them come?

*Explore Kink:* By exploring BDSM and different forms of kink, you can channel the open-mindedness that will allow the connection that Tantra is about. When you can put yourself in a vulnerable position, you are in a position to be opened, and this is a large part of Tantra. This could mean being blindfolded, getting whipped, or just sharing your fetishes; you can tap into some tantric sex principles just be making eye contact and breathing. When you have learned how to be vulnerable with your partner, the transformation will happen. You might cry when you deblock. This is all a part of Tantra even if it doesn't look like it.

*Talk While Having Sex:* According to Tantra, the sex, touching, and kissing is a great way to connect and the best way to help this connection is talking to your partner while doing everything. Instead of just guessing that your partner's moan during oral sex means they are enjoying it, step up your game and talk to your partner about what you like and don't like. Moaning is great, but tell them what you like about their technique. When we talk about our pleasure and give our partner praise, it makes them want to do more and builds trust and intimacy.

*Synchronize Your Breathing:* Stop whatever you are doing and take ten long, deep breaths. Did that make you feel better? Good. Take ten deep breaths before touching your partner to get yourself grounded. When things begin to get sexy, take the breathing a step further by synchronizing your breaths. These should be done facing your partner, so a sexual position like Lap Dance and look into each other's eyes. Follow the other's breathing until the sync up. If you can harmonize your breathing, this allows an energetic connection to happen especially if you are sitting with your genitals touching.

*Make a List of What Turns You On:* Tantra is friendly for beginners. It requires you to do some homework, but it is fun. Communication is the key to making the connection that Tantra is all about. You need to know what turns you on before you tell your partner what you want and need. During tantric sex exercises, each partner will write a list of what turns them on. After each partner has made theirs, they will exchange the lists and talk about what is on them. This activity can turn into a steamy brainstorming session, after all, it is dirty talk. It is a great opportunity to learn about your partner and yourself. Any kink from BDSM to role-playing can be tantric when done correctly.

*Masturbate:* This is great news. You don't need to have a partner to add Tantra to your life. Anybody can try Tantra simply by masturbating. If you are single, this is a great time to work on your desires, to breathe, being in the moment, and sexually explore yourself. Practicing Tantra when flying solo allows you to tune into yourself when you do have sex with a partner. If you have a partner and they don't want to explore Tantra, masturbating is a great way to put it in your life.

*Practice:* More clearly, practice without judging. It is so easy getting hung up on feeling discouraged or inadequate, but those are never productive. We judge ourselves and can't move forward. We can't or won't explore because we have decided that we suck. Treat Tanta like anything else you do like sweeping the floor or brushing your teeth. It isn't about doing it wrong or right. It's about finding and exploring what would happen. Practicing Tantra is more fun that brushing your teeth.

*How to End Your Session:* By now you are probably ready to have sex or not. If you don't want to just lay in each other's arms and share your feelings. If you are going to have sex, don't rush it. Let the penetration happen on its own without making an effort. Begin with shallow, slow thrusts and remain aware of your genitals, energies, and bodies. Guide the consciousness up and down the spine going between the heart and genitals. Notice the sensation going through your body. As you begin to move, let your genitals melt into an ecstatic and sensual dance. Take your time. Remember, Tantra is not about orgasm. It is a pleasure feast. If both of you are experiencing lots of pleasure, you are doing something right.

*Top Tantric Tip:* Slow down your breathing as you reach orgasm. Most people breathe quicker as the feel the orgasm coming on. They will tense, and they try to make it happen. Instead, relax the stomach and take deep, slow breaths into your stomach. Your orgasm will be more intense and last longer.

# The Seventh Chakra

The seventh chakra, which is also called the thousand-petal lotus chakra or Sahaswara, is located at the crown of the head. This chakra is where we receive our enlightenment and our connection to our spirituality. This is where we connect with our higher being, every other person on earth, and the divine energy that created everything within the universe.

When the seventh chakra is truly opened, you will soon realize that you are complete awareness. You are completely all expansive, undivided, and conscious. Just like a drop in the ocean, you are a piece of the ocean that encompasses every single aspect of it.

The seventh chakra is closely related to the following behavioral and psychological characteristics:

- Presence

- Bliss, ecstasy

- Connection with higher conscious states

- Liberate from limiting patterns, realization

- Limitless, connected with the formless

- Awareness and wisdom of the higher consciousness and what is sacred

- Consciousness

The lotus flower can be found in Buddhist and Hindu traditions. The plants are nurtured, grown, and emerges from muddy waters. The flower will bloom even when there isn't any clarity. Lotus has a beauty that stands out and is unique in its environment of monotony and lackluster vibrancy.

When this chakra unfurls, you will notice that you start to emerge out of the confines of your body, intellect, mind, and ego. You will even be able to push out of the individual soul that holds you to Samsara, the endless birth and rebirth cycle. You are no longer shackled to desire. White light will surround you, and you stand out among your murky surroundings.

This chakra is the center of positivity, happiness, inspiration, devotion, and trust. It will also give you a closer connection with yourself and a greater connection with the life force that is higher than your being. Because of this, it is very useful to have the chakra open.

If your crown chakra is out of balance you will notice some of the following:

- Closed-mindedness

- Materialism and greed

- Chronic headaches, migraines

- Obsessively attached to spiritual problems

- Chronic fatigue

- Feeling disconnected with your earthly and bodily matters

- Cynical regarding the sacred, disconnection with the spirit

- Mental fog and depression

- If your crown chakra is overactive, you may feel disconnected to your body

If your crown chakra is receiving too much energy you may experience:

- Sense of unearned accomplishment and elitism

- Frustration and boredom

- Endocrine or neurological disorders

- Sensitivity to sound and light

A seventh chakra that is unbalanced can also play a part in mental illnesses, sleep disorders, comas, and learning disabilities.

The goal of this chapter is to help you open your seventh chakra. At this point, you may be thinking that it sounds great and it may work for gurus and monks, but you're just an ordinary person. How are you supposed to be able to obtain something like that?

While you may have to work around the demands of your life and your busy mind, but reaching enlightenment isn't as hard to obtain as it may seem. A hard goal to work towards is living in a state of constant and pure awareness. So why not to work towards living with only moments of awareness? We've all had a few of those moments and different times. Think about times when you have felt unconditional love for something or someone, or maybe you have experienced some miracle.

Ways to achieve these moments is through daily silence, meditation, and prayer to increase spiritual connection. During these practices, you will experience what Sahaswara is. After you establish a regular daily practice of this kind of activities that help to connect you with your universal consciousness, you will start to see the growth of your spiritual awareness in your everyday life. You will notice that you consistently feel unconditional love. You'll notice that you are more forgiving, compassionate, and kind and you will have more humility. You will no longer live your life solely for yourself and desires. You will start to help others more because when you help others, you are also helping yourself.

The seventh chakra is mainly associated with the pituitary gland but is also related to the hypothalamus and pineal gland. The pituitary gland and hypothalamus work together to help keep your endocrine system regulated. Since the crown chakra is located at the top of the head, it is associated closely with the brain and much of the nervous system.

The colors white and violet are closely associated with the crown chakra, and its mantra sound is the very common and universal sound of OM. The best gems to wear or keep in your environment that can help align and open this chakra are sugilite, amethyst, and selenite. You can also use aromatherapy to help clear your seventh chakra. The scents lavender rose, and jasmine can help to calm an overactive crown chakra. You can use myrrh, frankincense, and sandalwood to stimulate and crown chakra that is underactive.

Remember, that in an energetic sense, the seventh and first chakras are very closely related because they are both extremities of the chakra system. Also, before you begin working with your crown chakra, you need to make sure that your root chakra is balanced first. You have to have a good foundation and a house before you can place on the roof. You have to work from the bottom up; you shouldn't start at the top.

While you can open the seventh chakra easily through silence, and it's the most important way to do so, there are also several other ways to help support and open this chakra.

There are two pranayama breathing practices that you can use before you begin your meditation; Kapalabhati, or skull shining breath, and Nadi Shodhana, or alternate nostril breathing.

While meditation is considered to be the best way to open and balance the crown chakra, many asanas can help to heal your seventh chakra. Inverted yoga asanas are also great to stimulate your seventh chakra; these include down dog and headstand. You can also try postures that bring the crown of the head into contact with the floor, like the fish pose. The following are also great:

- Supta Baddha Konasana or Reclining Bound Angle – This pose helps to stretch out the hips and stimulate the reproductive organs and kidneys while it balances and opens the crown chakra.

- Paschimottanasana or Seated Forward Bend – By allowing the shoulders and spine stretch, the seated posture helps heal, open, and balance the crown chakra while stimulating the kidneys, liver, and reproductive organs.

- Padmasana or Lotus – This post helps to stimulate the core and spine while also calming and balancing the crown chakra.

- Salamba Sarvangasana or Supported Shoulderstand – This helps to tone up the lower part of the body. This pose will help to calm and balance the seventh chakra as well as alleviate depression.

- Halasana or Plow – This inverted pose helps to stretch the shoulders and spine while it also balances and soothe the crown chakra.

- Salamba Sirsasana or Supported Headstand – This is an advanced pose that helps to nourish the head with blood and oxygen to help soothe, open, and balance the seventh chakra.

Adding a yoga routine to your lifestyle will not only help your chakra system but will help you benefit you it all aspects of your life. Asanas or yoga poses work by dispelling blockages and negativity to promote a healthy energy flow through the all the energy centers in the body. Also, when you are only focusing on one chakra, you are still helping all the others.

Some other great ways to open your crown chakra are to:

1. Visualize

   One way to open the crown chakra is to use visualization. Start by imagining a golden orb of light filling up your head. Watch as this orb starts to grow and expand. Imagine that it's growing your thoughts and filling your body with positivity. Picture a golden light streaming from the top of your head and connecting you with the universe above you. Notice how your head feels open and expanded. Notice the unity and oneness you feel with life. Notice how you are connected with the force of life that is bigger than you are. Use this affirmation: I'm connected with a life force that is bigger than me. Take note of how you feel with this connection. Also, remember that no matter where you are in your life and in your world, you will never be alone.

   As you picture this, you are helping the crown chakra to open up and connect you with a life force that is bigger than you are.

2. Get inspired

   Another great way to open the crown chakra is with inspiration. Think about a concert you have been to or the way you feel when you hear a song that you love. Think of how these things made you feel. If you enjoyed being at the concert or hearing the song you probably had a positive, open, inspired and uplifted feeling. These feelings are from and open crown chakra. You can listen to inspiring music, watch the sunset, read poetry, or take a walk through nature to help open your crown chakra. Anything that will bring inspiration to you will also help to open your crown chakra. Take a second now to think about the things that bring you inspiration. Start making sure that you find inspiration every day so that your crown chakra stays open.

3. Practice affirmations

Another crown chakra opening practice is to use inspiring affirmations. You can use this affirmation and repeat it quietly: "I am open and expanded. I expand my idea of what is possible. As I expand my idea of what is possible, I help to bring it in. I am open and expanded." Start to become aware of how expanded and open you feel at the top of your head. This is how it feels when your crown chakra is open. Repeat any inspiring affirmation that you want throughout your day so that you keep the crown chakra open.

As you have learned, having an opened crown chakra is an important and valuable tool. Try to implement these different practices every day so that you feel more connected to your greater life force, positivity, trust, and inspiration.

# Tantric Breathing

The way you breathe has a huge impact on your emotional and physical health. Tantra teaches you breathing techniques within its scriptures. Besides the fact that this breathing technique can help you spiritually, physically, and mentally, tantric breathing is also a great to detoxify your system.

A lot of people believe that you breath should come from the chest, but this isn't true. This is commonly believed within the physical fitness world. If you only breathe in your chest, it can cause many complications because the lungs are unable to expand completely which means they are not able to absorb oxygen correctly. The first thing most tantra teachers will tell their students is that chest breathing is unhealthy and shallow breaths.

Another problem with chest breathing is that the expanded chest is a way that men behave to show dominance and aggression. This look is a primitive response to danger, and its only real purpose it to make a person look larger and take up more space, making them appear more powerful. Because of this, when you constantly expand your chest to breathe, you're causing your body to release different kinds of stress hormones.

To be successful with tantra, it's important that you can unlearn your unhealthy breathing pattern, and learn the problem tantric breathing techniques. This is not an easy thing to do.

Another important part of tantric breathing is to help a person achieve multiple orgasms, without ejaculating. This allows you open the door to erotic ecstasy with the use of sexual continence while making love. This means that you will learn how to control your capacity and erotic sensitiveness.

It is believed that when a man ejaculates it will decrease, and possibly exhaust his sexual energy reserve. When you learn tantric breathing, this will decrease the amount of sexual energy that you expel as well as giving you a chance to experience multiple orgasms.

The breathing techniques effectiveness all depends on how often and frequently you practice the techniques. There are going to be people that have more sensibility and erotic energy, and that have better mental control.

Some men that choose to practice these techniques to achieve multiple, non-ejaculatory, orgasms will be able to do so in only a week's time. While others, who have weaker mental controls, while likely have to practice for a few months, or possibly years.

## Breath

Breath is an involuntary action of the human body, but it's important that you make it a conscious act. This means that we normally breathe without thinking and without changing the rhythm of the breath. If we did start doing that, if breathing became a more profound act, then we would influence and change our cardiac rhythm.

Take for example after you have been running your breath is superficially and rapid which causes your cardiac rhythm to become higher. If you slow your breath down, then the cardiac rhythm also slows.

When it comes to lovemaking, if your cardiac rhythm becomes high you are approaching ejaculation. This means that to control ejaculation you have to learn how to control your breath.

## Abdominal Breath

Newborn babies, unlike most adults, breathe from their abdomen. If you ever watch a sleeping baby, you will start to notice that their belly moves with every breath they take. With abdominal breathing, you fill your lungs completely with air, which then replaces all the stagnating residual air in your lungs with new fresh air.

This is the healthiest way for a person to breathe, but, unfortunately, we forget how to because of anxiety and stress. This causes our breath to become limited to the upper chest area, which means we only breathe from the clavicles or thorax.

Think about when you are happy, and you laugh. When this happens, you breathe abdominally. The exercise that follows will teach you how to actively breathe abdominally, just like you did when you were a baby and like you do when you laugh.

When you are practicing this breathing technique, make sure you breathe in through the nose so that the air is warmed and filtered in your nasal passages. Remember that whenever you breathe through your mouth, you are taking in cold, unfiltered air.

1. Begin by sitting straight up in your chair with the spine straight, your head up, and your feet flat on the floor.

2. Gently lay your hands on your belly button and relax your shoulders.

3. Breathe in through your nose and notice how your lower abdomen is filled with air. This should cause you belly button to push forward as the diaphragm is pushed down.

4. Allow the chest to relax when you exhale forcefully out of your mouth. The lower abdomen should be pulled inwards as if your belly button is being pulled into your spine. For men, they should notices how the testicles and penis are slightly pulled upwards.

5. Continue to repeats steps three and four 21 times.

With only a few minutes of abdominal breathing, every day will train your body to properly breathe, naturally, and even while you are asleep. This type of breathing during lovemaking helps to expand your erotic sensations.

You should continue to practice this every day so that your body doesn't forget how to breathe. This will help your sexual energy to circulate throughout your body and will help turn it into affectionate and volitional mental energy.

Abdominal breathing also helps to message all of the internal organs, and, for men, the prostate. It also helps to relieve the pressure that men feel when they don't ejaculate. When you don't learn how to sublimate this tension caused by sexual continence, you will notice that you fell more on edge, confused, and irritable. Abdominal breathing helps to alleviate these problems.

Another tantric breathing exercise is through the practice of Hatha yoga postures. This will also eliminate your energy noses and help energy to circulate throughout your body. If you notice that you are having problems with abdominal breathing, like a lot of people do, then you can try abdominal laughter.

This doesn't mean little giggle; abdominal laughter is the kind of laughter that causes your belly to shake. This is the kind of genuine laughter that you share with close friends. This is laughter that causes you belly to hurt from laughing too much and cause you to tear up. The pain is caused by the fact that you are using muscles that you don't use all that often.

To begin this exercise, sit in a comfortable chair, with your feet on the floor, and your spine straight. Gently place your hands on your stomach and think of all the moments in your life that has made you laugh the hardest. When you notice the laughter is beginning, allow it to take hold of your whole body until you feel your belly begin to vibrate.

It's healthy for you to laugh like this because it helps to relax your diaphragm, causes abdominal breathing, and creates a lot of good energy, which you will be able to use later on.

# Conclusion

Thank for making it through to the end of *Tantric Sex*. Let's hope it was informative and able to provide you with all of the tools you need to achieve your goals.

The next step is to try out some of the things that you have learned in this book. Make sure to get on the same page as your partner and talk about what you both are willing to try.